HOMEMADE HAND SANITIZER

An easy guide to make DIY Anti-bacterial and Anti-Viral Hand Sanitizers from Home

By

Scarlett Maci

© **Copyright 2020 by Scarlett Maci- All rights reserved.**

This document is geared towards providing exact and reliable information in regards to the topic and issue covered. The publication is sold with the idea that the publisher is not required to render accounting, officially permitted, or otherwise qualified services. If advice is necessary, legal or professional, a practiced individual in the profession should be ordered.

- From a Declaration of Principles which was accepted and approved equally by a Committee of the American Bar Association and a Committee of Publishers and Associations.

In no way is it legal to reproduce, duplicate, or transmit any part of this document in either electronic means or printed format. Recording of this publication is strictly prohibited, and any storage of this document is not allowed unless with written permission from the publisher. All rights reserved.

The information provided herein is stated to be truthful and consistent, in that any liability, in terms of inattention or otherwise, by any usage or abuse of any policies, processes, or directions contained within is the solitary and utter responsibility of the recipient reader. Under no circumstances will any legal responsibility or blame be held against the publisher for any reparation, damages, or monetary loss due to the information herein, either directly or indirectly.

Respective authors own all copyrights not held by the publisher.

The information herein is offered for informational purposes solely and is universal as so. The presentation of the information is without a contract or any guarantee assurance.

The trademarks that are used are without any consent, and the publication of the trademark is without permission or backing by the trademark owner. All trademarks and brands within this book are for clarifying purposes only and are owned by the owners themselves, not affiliated with this document.

Table of Contents

INTRODUCTION 6

CHAPTER 1: HOMEMADE SANITIZERS AND THEIR NEED 8

1.1 Introduction to Hand Sanitizers 8

1.2 Difference Between Sanitizer And Disinfectant 8

1.3 Purpose of Sanitizer: 10

1.4 Why Homemade Sanitizers Are Becoming Important? 11

CHAPTER 2: HOMEMADE SANITIZER RECIPES 12

2.1 What To Know Before Making DIY Homemade Sanitizer? 12

2.2 Ingredients Required For Making Sanitizer At Home 14

2.3 Instructions for the Formulation 16

2.4 Instructions for Gel Sanitizer 17

2.5 Scented Homemade Sanitizer 18

2.6 How to make Alcohol Free Homemade Sanitizers? 18

CHAPTER 3: BENEFITS OF MAKING SANITIZER AT HOME 20

3.1 The Advantages of Homebased industry of Sanitizers 20

3.2 Keep Yourself Clean Using Reliable Sources 22

CHAPTER 4: EFFECTIVENESS OF HOMEMADE SANITIZER 24

4.1 Homemade Sanitizer Are Effective To Kill Germs 24

4.2 Homemade Sanitizer Can Be Your Travel Cleaning Buddy. 26

CHAPTER 5: IS HOMEMADE SANITIZER SAFE? 29

5.1 Is Soap And Water Better Than Homemade Sanitizer? 29

5.2 FDA Regulations to Make a Sanitizer 30

5.3 Precautionary Measures For The Use Of Homemade Sanitizers 32

CONCLUSION 35

REFERENCES 36

Introduction

Homemade Sanitizers are easy to make products that are essential for cleanliness in today's world. We use the same pair of hands to feed, thereby transmitting the disease through the mouth, and add germs to our body. As we perform our daily duties, holding a clean hand or washing our hands frequently always or after picking up items or eventually placing your hands-on dirty surfaces isn't easy. We also need a safe and secure means, and by using sanitizers, we can have clean hands.

Properly scrubbing your hands with hand sanitizer is one of the best ways to stop the spread of viruses and germs, and to ensure you don't get sick yourself. But if you don't have access to soap and clean water, or if you're out and about and nowhere near a toilet, you're expected to carry hand sanitizer for health safety.

It is easy to make one's hand sanitizer. You've just got to be cautious not to screw things up. Be sure to sanitize the equipment you use for mixing correctly; otherwise, you might contaminate the whole thing. Homemade hand sanitizers are just as successful as anything you're purchasing if you're using the correct amount of alcohol. It is a perfect way to get consumers suffering from price gouging.

The recent pandemic is causing more havoc than our physical health. Our mental health is affected by the fact that people are lined up in stores to buy supplies to prevent the virus from spreading or taking hold first. Distilleries move in to help combat the scarcity of hand sanitizers by using the alcohol in their facilities to make their drug-based alternatives. Some pack it in small bottles while others allow people to carry the refills in their containers.

The shortages and buying restrictions have inspired people to use Facebook, Reddit, Pinterest for recipes, numerous forums, and even a pharmacy to make their hand sanitizer. But just because there are those recipes doesn't mean that you can adopt them.

Next, the Centers for Disease Control recommends that you wash your hands using a hand sanitizer unless you have access to water and soap. Second, experts advise that it's more difficult to make homemade hand sanitizer than it seems. If you don't have the right concentration, experts say you're going to end up with something that isn't successful, or it's too harsh, and that's a waste of ingredients.

There are significant variations between soap and water washing hands and cleaning them with a hand sanitizer. Knowing when to wash your hands and which approach to use will give you the best opportunity to avoid illness.

Chapter 1: Homemade Sanitizers and Their Need

Homemade hand sanitizer provides several advantages over handwashing with soap and water. Most importantly, they require less time than hand washing and are more accessible than sinks. Also, they are less irritating to the skin than soap and water. Some can even improve the condition of the skin.

1.1 Introduction to Hand Sanitizers

In 1966, Lupe Hernandez, a registered nurse in Bakersfield, California, invented the self-made sanitizers. When Hernandez was training to become a nurse, she found that a gel can be used to administer cleaning alcohol so that washing could take place without soap and water. In hand sanitizers, the alcohol destroys the germs and bacteria present on paws.

Hand sanitizer, also called hand antiseptic, hand rub, or hand rubbing agent applied to the hands to kill growing pathogens (organisms that cause disease). Usually, hand sanitizers come in the form of paste, gel, or liquid. Its use is recommended when soap and water are not enough for hand washing or when frequent hand washing interferes with the natural skin barrier (e.g., causing the skin to develop scaling or fissures). Although the efficacy of the hand sanitizer is subjective, it is used in a wide range of settings as a primary means of infection prevention, from day-care centers and schools to hospitals and health care facilities, and from supermarkets to cruise ships.

1.2 Difference Between Sanitizer And Disinfectant

The terms sanitize and disinfect tossed around a lot when you speak or read about cleaning, particularly when you tackle a deep clean. They are also used interchangeably in casual uses, although there is a significant difference between sanitizing and disinfecting. Understanding the difference between the two will influence the items you use to clean and how you use them, and it can mean having a healthier, cleaner position where you need it most.

Sanitization removes a virus or bacteria to a safe level, whereas disinfection destroys anything on a specified surface. Think of sanitizing as lowering germ levels on a surface, while disinfecting destroys them all. Sanitizing is a bit gentler than disinfecting, which can be useful and requires strong chemicals often.

So, when are you supposed to sanitize, and when do you disinfect? Sanitizing is better for surfaces that do not usually encounter highly hazardous bacteria. Those that are left without contact with potent chemicals: think of cooking equipment and food preparation surfaces or toys that children come into near contact with (or even bring into their mouths). Disinfecting is for the significant messes, particularly those that contain body fluids, blood, and the like. You'd clean a toilet or sink in household settings; disinfection is often commonly used in medical settings.

If it comes to choosing sanitizing vs. disinfecting, you'd like to use a more effective disinfecting agent than you would for sanitizing. Water and bleach solutions can be both a sanitizer and a disinfectant (in a lower concentration for the former, in a higher frequency for the latter), and they can be reasonably effective, efficient, so long as you follow the guidelines for contact time. On the other hand, cleaning vinegar is an ordinary cleaner, but it isn't a registered disinfectant or sanitizer, and can't kill dangerous bacteria.

If you're doing a regular, gentle cleaning as part of your checklist for cleaning, you're good with a mild cleaner and just sweep away dirt and grime. However, understanding the difference between sanitizing and disinfecting will help you decide when to take the heavy-duty cleaners out if you need anything more substantial. You should at least be confident you're tossing around correct vocabulary.

1.3 Purpose of Sanitizer:

People use their hands to write a report during the entire working day, shake hands with a new customer, open doors, and much more. All those behaviors expose hands to dangerous bacteria and germs. Most of the public is also aware of the need to use hand sanitizer when soap and water are not available. Although most households and workplaces have a steady supply of soap, a reasonably new change is the introduction of a hand sanitizer into the customer mentality and industry.

Hand sanitizers are thought to offer some of the advantages of handwashing to customers when handwashing isn't practical. Epidemiological studies have not identified the connection between manual sanitizer use and reduced disease, but some laboratory studies indicate that hand sanitizers help prevent infection by killing transient pathogenic bacteria.

Handwashing-whether performed with "antibacterial" soap, or simple soap-physically eliminates microorganisms from the skin, washing down the drain where microbes live. Hand sanitizers minimize rates of organisms by chemically destroying them much like disinfectants kill germs on surfaces throughout the world.

The extent of the handwashing effect is mainly a function of washing time and the use of the soap. Without soap washing, the hands are much less capable. Hand sanitizer efficacy is highest when applying a large amount of liquid to the sides. The application of a large amount of hand sanitizer guarantees an abundance of the active ingredient and increases the duration of chemical action until evaporation of the hand sanitizer.

1.4 Why Homemade Sanitizers Are Becoming Important?

Hand sanitizer has never been more popular, as it has been widely reported as one of the best ways to protect yourself on the go. When you and your loved ones are out shopping, traveling, or doing other public events, you're bound to feel like you need a quicker cure, particularly during the cold and flu season or the spread of more severe. You shouldn't wait until you get home to fight germs at your hands while you're out and about If water and soap is not available than use a hand sanitizer, containing at least 60 percent alcohol should be used. Hand sanitizer is a convenient and straightforward solution that is safe to travel with, which, according to the CDC, will minimize the number of microbes that germs on your hands. If hands cannot be washed with soap and water, store-bought, scientifically formulated hand sanitizers are a reliable next choice.

If you have trouble tracking down the store's hand sanitizer, then you can make your own. Making your DIY hand sanitizer is a natural process requiring just a few ingredients (although you can add a few more for extra benefit).

Chapter 2: Homemade Sanitizer Recipes

Some people could try to make it at home, due to a possible shortage of hand sanitizers in stores. Continue reading to learn more about homemade hand sanitizer, including risks, health, and official recommendations.

2.1 What To Know Before Making DIY Homemade Sanitizer?

Several experts offered insights into what precautionary steps to take, how you can be diligent in preventing yourself and others from catching the virus, and the best way to make your hand sanitizer using ingredients that you might already have at home.

The CDC stresses that while in some cases, "alcohol-based sanitizers will rapidly reduce the number of microbes on hands," they are not getting rid of every kind of germ. Additionally, if you intend to make your hand sanitizer, note that you need to calculate the ingredients precisely for the product to function. Else, more damage can be done than good.

Carl Fichtenbaum, an expert and professor of clinical medicine at the University of Cincinnati, tells Popular Mechanics that "It's not a bad idea" when it comes to DIY hand sanitizer. He also emphasizes the value of product calculation for efficacy.

"When you can make a sanitizer with the correct isopropyl alcohol or ethanol content—60 percent or more — it will probably work well," says Fichtenbaum.

Many of the online recipes we've seen do use this as the main ingredient, while others recommend using essential oils as the main ingredient instead of alcohol.

Many papers or blog posts apply to guidelines issued by the WHO. Only question? These instructions are not intended for the average DIY enthusiast. They include a range of products, such as an alcoholometer and vast quantities of highly flammable ingredients that you are unlikely to have around.

Commercial hand sanitizers also have emollients for keeping your skin soft and reducing any damage. Significant, because dry and damaged skin may increase the risk of viruses entering the skin through cuttings. Although many DIY recipes recommend adding aloe vera for its moisturizing properties, you run the risk of diluting the alcohol concentration if you don't get the right amount, rendering it ineffective.

Online, people will find different recipes for hand sanitizers. The WHO recommends using only the ingredients specified in its approved recipe for the hand sanitizer. Other ingredients that people can find online but should not use include:

• Russian usually only contains 40% alcohol. The CDC recommends hand sanitizers that contain alcohol of at least 60 percent. Besides, the FDA has approved the use of USP grade ingredients for manufacturing hand sanitizers only.

• Bleach is an active surface disinfectant when adequately prepared. Always obey the package instructions and use it carefully, because bleach can burn or irritate the skin.

Hand sanitizers based on bleach are not recommended for prolonged use, because they can damage the skin over time.

• Many different industries use silver and silver nanoparticles for their antimicrobial properties, such as the healthcare and food industries. Since silver ions have excellent antimicrobial properties and no significant human consequences, researchers report extensive use of silver-based products. Some bacteria which cause human infections to have developed resistance to silver's antimicrobial effects.

The environmental hazards of using silver as an antimicrobial agent are still not identified to researchers. Because some microorganisms that develop resistance to silver-based antimicrobial products, it is recommended that people avoid using them in homemade hand sanitation.

As easy as making your hand sanitizer, you should be aware that high quantity rubbing alcohol will harm your skin. Make sure that you stick to the 2:1 ratio to keep the alcohol level below 60%. You may also use gloves with the hand moisturizer when mixing and following up sanitization.

2.2 Ingredients Required For Making Sanitizer At Home

The most active part of this hand sanitizer recipe is alcohol, which must constitute at least 60 percent of the liquid to be an effective disinfectant. The recipe asks for 99 percent isopropyl alcohol (rubbing alcohol) or ethanol (grain alcohol, 90 percent -95 percent most commonly available). Since they are poisonous, please do not use any other forms of alcohol (e.g. methanol, butanol) Also, if you use a product that contains a lower level of alcohol (e.g. 70 percent alcohol) then you have to raise the amount of alcohol in the recipe, or it won't be as successful.

- **Essential Oils in Hand Sanitizer**

In order to add fragrance to your hand sanitizer, the essential oil you use can also help to protect you against germs. Thyme and clove oil, for example, have antimicrobial properties. If you are using antimicrobial oils, use just one or two drops, as these oils appear to be very strong and may irritate your skin. Other oils, including chamomile or lavender, can help soothe your skin.

- **Tea Tree Oil Has Antimicrobial Properties.**

A few drops can be used in the recipe, but it is essential to remember that even though it is diluted, many people are sensitive to this oil.

- **Substitutions**

Alcohol is the main ingredient in the hand sanitizer, and an aloe vera gel can be substituted. The aloe gel helps to shield the hands from the drying effects of alcohol. It is, essentially, a humectant, this means keeping in moisture helps. Many humectants that may be used as an alternative to aloe include glycerin or hand lotion.

However, maintaining the alcohol in the final product at least 60 percent is still necessary.

If you can't find alcohol, washing your hands with soap and water is the safest choice, rather than attempting a homemade recipe for a hand sanitizer.

- **Operating with 70% alcohol:**

Rubbing alcohol and ethanol from a pharmacy appears to be either 90-99% alcohol, or 70% alcohol, respectively. With 70 percent alcohol, you can clean your hands, but it is very small you can add to it (perhaps a few drops of essential oil) to enhance the smell or texture. Mixing 70 percent of alcohol with other ingredients dilutes the alcohol, making it possible to slip below the CDC's prescribed 60 percent alcohol.

- **Secure your hands**

As alcohol dries the skin and natural oils strings. To keep the skin in top condition, follow a hand sanitizer (or hand wash) with a decent lotion. Damaged skin contains tiny cracks that trap bacteria and viruses and make them more challenging to remove. Try to keep the amount of alcohol in the hand sanitizer about 60-70 percent (as in this recipe) if you have sensitive skin since a higher concentration can irritate.

2.3 Instructions for the Formulation

The WHO has a detailed guide on how to make your hand sanitizer the only thing is that you will end up with a lot of it if you obey these directions. Like, of that, precisely 2.6 gallons. If you want to make enough to last you, your family and all your friends, you will probably. But if you want to keep things smaller, we have customized the dimensions for you.

- 1 cup of 99 percent isopropyl alcohol
- 1 tablespoon of 3 percent hydrogen peroxide
- 1 teaspoon of 98 percent glycerin
- 1/4 cup (or 65 milliliters) of sterile distilled or boiling cold water

1- Pour the Alcohol into a medium-sized jar with a spout.

The percentages on the isopropyl alcohol labels contribute to the concentration of alcohol in them. When you have 99.8 percent, you are dealing with almost pure alcohol, while 70 percent means that the bottle is just over two-thirds alcohol, and the remainder is water. Some formulations have attempted to modify this to use 91% or even 70% of isopropyl alcohol. But these amounts of alcohol can make a finished product which does not comply with the advice of the Centers for Disease Control and Prevention to use hand sanitizers.

2- Add the hydrogen peroxide.

3- Apply the glycerin, then whisk. This element is thicker than both alcohol and hydrogen peroxide, so mixing it will take some stirring. For this, you can use a clean spoon or, if your jar has a lid, you can put it on and well shake it.

4- Weigh water and pour it in. Measure and add 1/4 of a cup of distilled or boiling cold water to the mixture.

5- Sanitize the spray bottles and pour the sanitizer into your mouth.

Sprinkle some of your leftover alcohol into your bottles and let them stay until the alcohol evaporates.

2.4 Instructions for Gel Sanitizer

Following are the ingredients to make gel homemade sanitizer:

- 1 cup of 91 percent alcohol isopropyl
- 1/2 cup of aloe vera gel (natural or store-bought)
- 15 drops of tea tree oil (or other essential antibacterial liquid)

1. Load the alcohol into a medium vessel with pouring sputum. Some online recipes use vodka rather than isopropyl alcohol, but most vodkas do not have enough alcohol to be successful. Note: The use of more than 91 percent diluted isopropyl alcohol can result in a weaker hand sanitizer that does not reach the 60 percent requirement of the CDC.

2. Measure the aloe vera gel and pour it over. Alcohol on your skin can be rough, but using aloe is a safe way to mitigate the impact and keep your hands clean. If you want to keep things safe, you can use aloe vera gel straight from the plant without worrying that something will go wrong — the alcohol will serve as a preservative. You will need to have in mind, though, that natural aloe gel is thicker than its store-bought equivalent and thus affects the final product differently it will make your hand sanitizer stickier, meaning you will need to rub your hands more often to absorb it completely.

3. Stir in the hot oil. Naturally, tea tree oil is antibacterial, so it makes sense to use it here. But if you're not a fan of his scent, you can use essential oil, such as lavender, lemongrass, or eucalyptus.

4. Stirring won't be enough to thoroughly combine all ingredients. Get a whisk and beat a homogeneous gel with the hand sanitizer.

5. Sanitize the spray bottles, then pour the sanitizer into your side. Sprinkle some of your leftover alcohol into your bottles and let them stay until the alcohol evaporates.

2.5 Scented Homemade Sanitizer

If you love natural oils, you will love this.

- **Aloe vera gel**
- **Rubbing alcohol**
- **Cinnamon essential oil**
- **Tea tree essential oil**
- **Dissolved water**

1. Start with 1/4 cup aloe vera gel emptying into a small mixing bowl.
2. Last, add a spoonful of rubbing spirits.
3. Add ten drops of essential oil made from cinnamon.
4. And ten drops of essential oil from the Tea tree.
5. Finally, add a spoonful of distilled water and stir.
6. Using a funnel to pour the hand sanitizer into a container until all the ingredients are mixed, and the consistency is smooth.

2.6 How to make Alcohol Free Homemade Sanitizers?

As far as alcohol-free sanitizers are concerned, we can use the following:

- 2-ounce spray bottle
- 5 drops of vitamin E oil (optional, this makes for soft hands!)
- 5 drops of essential lemon oil

- 5 drops of essential orange oil
- 5 drops of essential tea tree oil
- Distilled (or at least washed, processed, and place the sprayer firmly on and shake well to combine for 15-20 seconds.

Open the bottle and fill in water to the rim. Replace sprayer, then shake for 15-20 seconds again. To apply: vigorously shake the container to reincorporate the essential oils, then spray liberally on your hands if you feel they need a bit of a deep clean. Clean your hands until dry.

- **Essential oil disclaimer:**

This recipe uses what is generally considered safe essential oils, but please bear in mind that while completely natural, all essential oils are powerful plant compounds to which you and your family (including your pets) may respond.

Always use essential oils undiluted or take essential oils internally (diluted or undiluted) without a professional's advice, and please learn about the potential side effects of each oil form before using it.

In the first trimester of pregnancy, limit the use of essential oils (diluted or undiluted) on small babies and on those with serious allergies to plants from which the oils are obtained.

So, if you see any reactions inside yourself, your family, or your pets, immediately stop using your essential oil products, so contact a medical professional.

- **High-proof grain alcohol use:**

The use of high-proof grain alcohol (Ever clear) in this recipe can be very hand drying.

Chapter 3: Benefits of Making Sanitizer At Home

In a struggle to survive during the recession, small companies are turning their models up. Many distilleries have begun producing hand sanitizer gel in the UK. According to a BBC study, a micro-distillery in Bristol, is making 100ml bottles and selling them to people in exchange for a donation. Manager Danny Walker aims to bring it to hospitals too. Pai Skincare, based in West London, has also turned to manufacture the hand sanitizer, announcing its first batch on Thursday. According to foundress Sarah Brown, the product took two weeks to create, rather than the normal 18 months.

3.1 The Advantages of Homebased industry of Sanitizers

Home-based company shall be any company where the primary office is situated in the home of the owner. You don't need to buy the house, but you need to operate a business from the same premises that you live in to make the business home business. Though we expect home-based business owners to operate at home, this is not always the case. Computer engineers, truckers, and interior decorators are just three examples of people who may operate home-based businesses but must travel to provide their services.

There are several things while running a home business that attracts people to it, especially when it comes to spending and tax savings.

Private liberty: When you're used to wasting hours in traffic every day to and from work, two of the most exciting benefits of starting a home-based company are your newfound independence and the recovery of lost time.

According to the US, the average American spends 348 hours of commuting per year. Suddenly, you have some extra hours with a home-based company to regain control of your personal life. Plus, there's no bosses, no dress code, no fixed schedule of work, and no maneuverable bureau politics. What you need is personal motivation, consistency, and the ability to manage time.

You get to keep the money that you are making. It is a basic principle: the harder you are working, the more money you can make. The potential of your earning is directly proportional to your results, so you don't need to wait for a promotion or a raise. You are working more and delivering better. You'll save gas and food money too. Home lunch planning is more cost-effective and provides a good break in the workday.

Gain potential: Starting your own home-based business with so many businesses and sectors in a recession means you can build your own income-producing opportunities.

In certain sectors, good job prospects can be scarce, and promotional incentives within major companies are also diminishing.

Danger less: Running a business from home requires even less cash for start-ups than a freestanding business or even a franchise. And once the company is up and running, managing it is cheaper and simpler than having a separate company place.

Tax incentives: There is a range of tax benefits of getting your home and office under one roof. As company expenses, you can subtract a portion of the operating and depreciation expenses of your house. It can be a percentage of your mortgage, income taxes, insurance, electricity, and/or household maintenance expenses.

Time for family and friends: This is particularly important for parents of school-age children: when they return, you will see the children off to school and be home on most days. Sometimes, if someone's sick, leaving the desk in your home is better than leaving one in the office of another.

Less exhaustion: Juggling the pressures of work and family is a little less difficult when you know you can stay home to care for a sick child and simply set your own timetable.

Professional development incentives: Having your own boss gives you the ability to wear loads of hats: sales director, marketing specialist, consultant, manager of business growth, and more. This gives you knowledge and experience in all aspects of running a company, which in effect makes you marketable even more.

Growing efficiency: Now that you no longer have to budget time and energy for commuting or a series of pointless meetings, you will have far more time and energy to make the success of your company.

An innovative springboard: Launching your home can be an opportunity for you to put your interests and hobbies into being and create a cash-generating platform for your unique and creative talents.

3.2 Keep Yourself Clean Using Reliable Sources

Good skin pH is about 5.5, which is slightly acidic but has a much higher pH in most traditional hand sanitizers — trusted Source, often as high as 11. "If the pH of the skin is too high, the body will produce excess sebum to fight back and restore its normal pH.

However, the residue from the sanitizers ensures that the destructive pH is preserved, "says independent beauty chemist David Pollack. "The end result is skin may get too oily. If that's not bad enough, the residue of the sanitizers emulsifies or attaches to the lipid matrix of the skin. "

But the advantage here is that if you're going to make your own sanitizer, then you're going to make it according to your needs, which will help you clean and keep you healthy.

Chapter 4: Effectiveness of Homemade Sanitizer

Hand sanitizers can be used in nursing homes and hospitals exits, and in many public washrooms. We all know the importance of proper handwashing to reduce the insecure transmission of the germs. There are times, though, when there is no access to soap and water or insufficient time for thorough washing.

4.1 Homemade Sanitizer Are Effective To Kill Germs

Waterless hand sanitizer provides some benefits over the soap and water hand cleaning.

Where organic matter (dirt, food, or other material) is visible on hands; they are not successful.

Waterless hand sanitizer benefits:

- Take less time than hand washing
- Work rapidly to destroy microorganisms on the hands
- Are more available than sinks
- Minimize bacterial counts on the sides
- Do not encourage antimicrobial resistance
- Are less harmful to the skin than soap.
- Some will also boost skin condition.

Anyone who has been in the play area of a child has experienced this. As the kids get off the play equipment, the mothers reach into their bag to get their hand sanitizer. To remove the germs that have been transmitted to her face, each child gets a dab of sanitizer to rub into her hands. The idea is this approach will keep the children safer, and their families.

- **How much is it you can use?**

Place a small volume, the size of your thumbnail, on the palm of your hand to use hand sanitizers efficiently, and rub it over your whole side, including your nailbeds. If the gel evaporates completely in under Fifteen seconds, you haven't used enough stuff.

- **Limitations:**

Not all hand sanitizer is produced equal. Look for active ingredients in the bottle. The quality of alcohol may be in the form of ethyl alcohol, ethanol, or isopropanol. Those are all suitable types of alcohol. Be sure that whatever form of alcohol is mentioned, its concentration varies between 60 and 95 percent. To be successful, the alcohol content of less than 60 percent is not enough.

- **Doesn't cut alcohol by grime.**

If the alcohol in the sanitizer must work, all dirt, blood, and soil must first be cleaned away or washed away. In these cases, it is advised to hand-wash with soap and water.

Hand sanitizers are not cleaning agents and are not meant as a substitute for soap and water but as an extension habit. Sanitizers are typically used in combination with regular handwashing.

Using hand sanitizers is a practice that can help keep all of us exposed to fewer germs and can thus reduce our risk of becoming sick. Whether you're on the playground, using someone else's machine, or visiting a hospital mate, take the time to rub a few on your fingertips. It represents a simple step towards a safe winter season.

During the peak respiratory virus season [around November to April], the portable hand sanitizers do have a function as they make it much easier to clean your hand.

It's much easier to wash your hands when you are sneezing than using a hand sanitizer, particularly when you're outdoors or in a vehicle. The hand sanitizers are much more convenient, and people are more likely to clean their hands, so this is better than not washing at all.

According to the Centers for Disease Control (CDC), it must be used correctly for hand sanitizer to be successful. That involves using the right amount (read the label to see how much you can use it), then rubbing it on all hand surfaces until your hands are warm. Should not dry your hands after applying or wash them. There is no evidence of dangerous hand sanitizers dependent on alcohol and other antimicrobial materials. Theoretically, they may contribute to antibacterial resistance. This is the most widely cited explanation of why people argue against using hand sanitizers. But that wasn't confirmed. No evidence of resistance to alcohol-based hand sanitizers has been identified at the hospital. While no studies are suggesting that hand sanitizers certainly pose a threat, there is also no proof that they are doing a better job of protecting you against harmful bacteria than soap. And even in hospitals or when you can't get to a sink, hand sanitizers have their place, washing with soap and warm water is almost always a better option.

4.2 Homemade Sanitizer Can Be Your Travel Cleaning Buddy.

Occasionally when you need it most, you can't find a commercial hand sanitizer in store. In some instances, washing your hands thoroughly in warm soapy water is more successful than using the hand sanitizer. Though, it isn't always easy to wash your hands with soap while you are traveling on flights or public transport. In this case, the hand sanitizer is a reasonable substitute. In travel size packets, you can take hand sanitizer into an airplane in your hand luggage.

Steps to Make DIY Hand Sanitizer Gel for Travel:

- Take two parts 91 percent rubbing alcohol (or stronger)
- Take 1-part aloe vera gel
- Mix in a cup
- Fill a travel squeezable bottle smaller than 3.4 oz or 100 ml

Steps to Make DIY Hand Sanitizer Spray for Travel:

- Take rubbing alcohol with a 75 percent minimum alcohol level
- Add 1.5 ml glycerol to 98.5 ml rubbing alcohol
- Mix in a bowl together.
- Use a fuel to fill a travel size pump spray bottle that is smaller than 3.4 oz or 100 ml
- Make sure the spray bottle has a cap to avoid unintended pump pressing

Know hand sanitizers are less effective when the hands are greasy, sticky, or dirty. Hand sanitizer isn't a replacement for soap and water to wash your hands when you get the opportunity. Many health experts aren't advocating making your sanitizer. This is mostly because they're afraid you'll end up with an unsuccessful drug. Even if you have a store-bought hand sanitizer, hand washing is a must. When you carry your homemade sanitizer onto a flight in your hand luggage, it would need to be in a container of travel size below 3.4 oz or 100 ml. Don't fill the bottle up to the top you need to clear some room for the liquid to expand or contract due to air pressure changes. Since hand sanitizer is a liquid, you do need to pack it inside your clear toiletries bag for quarter plastic. Some people prefer to use a pump-dispenser jar. If you want a bottle like this, then make sure it has a cap to avoid spilling the liquid when it's in your pocket, other people have used bottles like a roll-on deodorant with rolling ball dispenser.

Your best choice could be your old empty travel-size hand sanitizer bottle, so if empty, don't throw it away. You may have read that alcohol is banned on planes by more than 70% percentage. That still holds for alcoholic drinks. Without question, you can take rubbing alcohol, which is more durable than 70%. You can make your hand sanitizer that is as good as a hand sanitizer purchased from a pharmacy. Nonetheless, hand sanitizer alone might not be the only way to avoid picking up germs while at airports or riding in flights. A sanitizer product is just an instrument in your toolkit. You should undoubtedly have antibacterial wipes in your flight packing list too.

These can be used to clean off the tray table and armrest. Try waking up early and going on the day's first flight if necessary. Aircraft are typically washed and disinfected overnight; the first flight of the day is when the plane is mostly clean. When you are using a hand sanitizer, handwashing with soap and warm water is always necessary. Wash your mouth, if you have the chance. Viruses are also spread by coughing and sneezing. It doesn't matter that how clean your hands are if you sit next to someone throwing a virus droplet out into the open. I will also pack pocket tissues not only for you, but if you end up sitting next to someone who doesn't sneeze or cough into the fabric. Any of your issues you may offer them.

Chapter 5: Is Homemade Sanitizer Safe?

Hands have the most interaction with other people, things, and our selves think how much you casually touch your face during the day. And while head-to-toe hygiene is a high priority for so many people, there is also an extreme emphasis on keeping the hands clean when it comes to preventing disease-carrying germs from spreading. Hand sanitizer has become a staple, even on keychains, in purses, pockets — and for a good reason.

5.1 Is Soap And Water Better Than Homemade Sanitizer?

Niket Sonpal, an internist, gastroenterologist, and adjunct professor at Touro College in New York, agrees that it may sometimes be the most convenient option: "The benefit of a hand sanitizer is the opportunity to combat germs when water and soap are not immediately available." Sonpal adds that hand sanitizers are efficient in neutralizing specific pathogens, viruses, and bacteria but not everything.

"Hand sanitizers are active against all forms of viruses except norovirus, which causes some form of diarrhea," explains Linda Anegawa, an internist based in Hawaii. They are, therefore, not a complete prophylactic though indeed serving a useful function. "Sanitizers often do not protect against some forms of bacteria, including one named C. difficile, which causes antibiotic overuse diarrhea." Athanasios Melisiotis, a Penn Medicine physician at the University of Pennsylvania, points out some other possible hand sanitizer downsides: "Some hand sanitizers can leave a residue where some users feel sticky or unpleasant," he says. "Hand sanitizers are nice and more convenient in a pinch, but ultimately soap and water are better."

- **Is Homemade Sanitizer Working?**

Hand sanitizer dependent on alcohol is user friendly, quick, and always easy to find. Although there's an excellent way to use hand sanitizer to get the most out of it, knowing when using it might not be the best option is probably more important. Hand sanitizer will help destroy bacteria, but it does not work on all germs and can do little with other substances that might be on your hands. There was no work about what they did and did not do when sanitizers first came out, but that has changed. There is a need to do more research, but scientists are learning more all the time.

Isopropyl alcohol (rubbing alcohol), a related type of alcohol (ethanol or n-propanol), or a mixture of both, is the active ingredient in hand sanitizers. Alcohols have long been known to destroy microbes by breaking down their protective outer protein layer and disrupting their metabolism. Evidence indicates, according to the CDC, that hand sanitizer removes germs as well as soap and water washing your hands – unless your hands are dirty or greasy.

Many scenarios when using a hand sanitizer may be acceptable include when you're driving public transportation, shaking hands, or holding an object, after holding a shopping cart, etc.

5.2 FDA Regulations to Make a Sanitizer

The U.S. Food and Drug Administration (FDA) released a final regulation intended to ensure better that over the counter (OTC) hand sanitizers are safe and efficient for those who rely on them.

The law states that all active ingredients that are sold under the FDA's OTC Drug Review are not approved to be used in OTC hand sanitizers, officially known as topical consumer antiseptic rub products, intended for waterless use. The final rule also attempts to ensure that the health and efficacy evaluations and determinations rendered by the agency for consumer antiseptic rub active ingredients are accurate, up-to-date, and accurately reflect existing scientific knowledge and that patterns of use. "Our action today is aimed at encouraging customers to be assured that the over-the-counter hand sanitizers they are using are safe and successful when they do not have access to soap washing water," said Janet Woodcock, MD, director of the FDA Drug Evaluation and Research Centre.

"In today's final rule, we finalized the previous FDA decision that active ingredients, including triclosan and benzethonium chloride, are not suitable for approval for use in consumer antiseptic rubbers under the FDA's OTC Drug Review.

We have reaffirmed our need for more data on three other active ingredients, including ethyl alcohol, the most widely used element in hand sanitizers, to assist the agency in ensuring that such items are safe and efficient for customers to use daily. We believe that the industry has made substantial strides in collecting data, and we will continue to provide the public with updates on the quality of this data collection. "Consumer antiseptic hand sanitizers offer a convenient option when handwashing with plain soap and water is not available.

Millions of Americans use regular, often several times a day, antiseptic rubbers to help eliminate bacteria on their palms.

As per CDC washing hands with regular soap and running water is one of the most effective steps people may take to stop getting sick and prevent diseases from spreading to others.

In the absence of water and soap, the CDC suggests using alcohol- hand sanitizer that contains at least one percent alcohol. The FDA is aware that manufacturers and pharmacies continue to sell a minimal number of generic hand sanitizers containing benzethonium chloride but have stopped the sale of triclosan-based hand sanitizers.

Pharmaceutical products that contain any unauthorized active ingredients may require prior marketing approval under a new drug application or abbreviated new drug application. The final rule completes a series of rulemaking steps to assess if such ingredients are safe and appropriate for their intended uses in the FDA's continuing review of OTC antiseptic active ingredients.

5.3 Precautionary Measures For The Use Of Homemade Sanitizers

1- Alcohol gel will catch fire and create a transparent blue flame. It is because the gel contains flammable alcohol. Many hand sanitizers gels due to a high concentration of water or moisturizing agents may not produce this effect. Alcohol rub users are advised to rub their hands until dry to reduce the risk of burning, which means the flammable alcohol has evaporated. Fire departments recommend that refills should be kept away from heat sources or open flames for alcohol-based hand sanitizers with cleaning supplies.

2- Research indicates that by removing beneficial microorganisms that are naturally present on the skin, alcohol hand sanitizers pose little risk.

3- Alcohol may remove the skin of the outer layer of oil, however, which can have adverse effects on the skin's barrier function.

Research also indicates that disinfecting hands with an antimicrobial detergent contributes to greater destruction of skin barriers compared to alcohol solutions, indicating an increased loss of skin lipids.

4- Food and Drug Administration (FDA) regulates hand-held antimicrobial soaps and sanitizers as over the-counter drugs (OTCs), since they are intended for topical antimicrobial use to avoid human disease. The FDA requires strict labeling to notify customers of the correct use of this OTC drug and to prevent risks, including informing adults not to drink, not to use in the eyes, to keep children out of reach, and to encourage children to use it only under adult supervision.

5-As per the American Association of Poison Control Centers, there were near reports of ingestion of hand sanitizers in. If swallowed, hand sanitizers based on alcohol can cause alcohol poisoning in infants. But the U.S. Centers for Disease Control recommends using hand sanitizer for children to encourage good health, under supervision, and recommends parents packing hand sanitizer for their children while traveling, to prevent their dirty hands contracting illness.

6-Incidents of people consuming the gel have been recorded in prisons and hospitals where alcohol intake is not tolerated to become intoxicated, leading to its removal from some establishments.

7-Non-alcohol-related, the FDA announced in April that it was seeking more scientific evidence focused on hand sanitizer health.

Emerging research also indicates that systemic exposure (full body exposure as shown by identification of antiseptic ingredients in the blood) is higher than commonly believed for at least some health care antiseptic active ingredients, and current evidence poses possible questions about the consequences of prolonged everyday human exposure to such antiseptic active ingredients. This may include alcohol- and triclosan-containing hand antiseptic products.

Conclusion

Hand Sanitizers are the best replacement for cleaning when soap and water is not available. However, they will be valid only for germs. Making a sanitizer at home is a do able task but keeping in view the concentrations of raw materials. Moreover, it is always better to use soap and water when available as using homemade sanitizer may be not effective in some cases like removing dirt. You can create different type of sanitizers at home as per your need and that will be beneficial for promoting home based industry as well. These homemade sanitizers will be according to our needs. Also, it is important to keep in mind about the usage of sanitizers and the precautions after their usage.

Hand sanitizer should not be used instead of soap and water when: cleaning is convenient Your hands are greasy or dirty You have chemicals on your hands You may have been exposed to infectious agents that are not destroyed by a hand sanitizer. It is important to wash your hands after you have used the toilet. It is safe to wash your hands vigorously with warm water and soap for seconds.

References

Introduction to Hand Sanitizers | Microchem Laboratory. (2020). Retrieved 27 March 2020, from **https://microchemlab.com/information/introduction-hand-sanitizers**

If You Don't Know the Difference Between Sanitizing and Disinfecting, You Might Not Be Cleaning Properly. (2020). Retrieved 27 March 2020, from **https://www.realsimple.com/home-organizing/cleaning/more-techniques/sanitize-vs-disinfect**

Introduction to Hand Sanitizers | Microchem Laboratory. (2020). Retrieved 27 March 2020, from **https://microchemlab.com/information/introduction-hand-sanitizers**

The role of hand sanitizer in infection control. (2020). Retrieved 27 March 2020, from **https://www.cleanlink.com/cleanlinkminute/details.aspx?id=23975**

hand sanitizer | Definition, Ingredients, Types, & Facts. (2020). Retrieved 27 March 2020, from **https://www.britannica.com/topic/hand-sanitizer**

Sanitizer, D. (2020). DIY Hand Sanitizer - Lexi's Clean Kitchen. Retrieved 27 March 2020, from **https://lexiscleankitchen.com/diy-hand-sanitizer/**

U.S. Food and Drug Administration. 2020. FDA Issues Final Rule On Safety And Effectiveness Of Consumer Hand Sanitizers. [online] Available at: https://www.fda.gov/news-events/press-announcements/fda-issues-final-rule-safety-and-effectiveness-consumer-hand-sanitizers.

www.ingramcontent.com/pod-product-compliance
Lightning Source LLC
Chambersburg PA
CBHW050307220526
45465CB00002B/856